OYA

IFÁ AND THE SPIRIT OF THE WIND

AWO FÁ'LOKUN FATUNMBI
OMO AWO FATUNMISE, ILE IFE,
BABALAWO ÈGBÈ IFÁ, ODE REMO,
OLÚWO ILÉ ÒRÚNMÌLÁ OSHUN, OAKLAND, CA

OYA; Ifa and the Spirit of the Tracker
By Awo Fa'lokun Fatunmbi

© ORIGINAL PUBLICATIONS 1993

ISBN: 0-942272-34-X

Original Publications
P.O. Box 236
Old Bethpage, New York 11804-0236
(888) OCCULT-1

www.OCCULT1.com

Printed in the United States of America

ACKNOWLEDGEMENTS

The material in this book is primarily based on oral instruction from the elders of *Ifá* in Ode Remo, Ogun State, Nigeria and Ile Ife, Oshun State, Nigeria. In appreciation for their time, patience and loving concern for my training and spiritual guidance I say: *A dúpé Ègbè Ifá* Ode Remo, *Babalawo* Adesanya Awoyade, *Babalawo* Babalola Akinsanya, *Babalawo* Saibu Lamiyo, *Babalawo* Odujosi Awoyade, *Babalawo* Olu Taylor, *Babalawo* Abokede Aralbadan, *Babalawo* Biodun Debona, *Babalawo* Oluwasina Kuti, *Babalawo* Afolabi Kuti, *Babalawo* Fagbemi Fasina, *Babalawo* Oropotoniyan and all the members of *Egbe Apetebi Ode Remo*.

Additional material in this book is based on instruction from the elders of Ile Ife, Oshun State, Nigeria. In appreciation to them I say: *A dúpé Awon Ifá* Fatunmise *Ègbè Ifá Ilé Ife, Jolofinpe* Falaju Fatunmise, *Babalawo* Ganiyu Olaifa Fatunmise, *Babalawo* Awoleke Awofisan Lokore, *Babalawo* Ifaioye Fatunmise, *Babalawo* Ifanimowu Fatunmise, *Babalawo* Ifasure Fatunmise, *Babalawo* Adebolu Fatunmise and all the members of *Egbe Apetebi Awon Fatunmise*.

A special thank you to the members of *Ilé Òrúnmìlà Oshun* for their continuing support and understanding: *Olori Yeye Aworo* Timi Lade, *Apetebi Orunmila, Iya l'Orisha* Oshun Miwa (Luisah Teish), *Eko'fa Iya l'Orisha* Omijinka, *Iya l'Orisha Iya* Oshun Iya Oshogbo, *Iya l'Orisha* Shango Wenwa, Nzinga Denny, Earthea Nance, Vance Williams, Blackberri, Salim Abdul-Jelani, Rebecca Schiros, Carol Lanigan, Zena Attig, Thisha, Rose Schadt, Xochipala Maes Valdez, Dee Orr, Nina Heft, Isoke, Luis Mangual and Earl White. A grateful thanks to *Awo* Medahochi and *Iya* Omolade.

A final thank you to Maureen Pattarelli for her work in editing this manuscript. *Orunmila a buru, a boye, a bosise.*

Awo Fá'lokun Fatunmbi
Oakland, CA

TABLE OF CONTENTS

INTRODUCTION

Oya is the Spirit of the Wind in the West African religious tradition called "*Ifá*". The word *Oya* is the name given to describe a complex convergence of Spiritual Forces that are key elements in the *Ifá* concept of change. Those Spiritual Forces that form the foundation of *Oya's* role in the Spirit Realm relate to the movement between dynamics and form as it exits throughout the Universe. According to *Ifá*, dynamics and form represent the polarity between the Forces of expansion and contraction. Together these Forces create light and darkness, which in turn sustains and defines all that is. According to *Ifá*, it is the interaction between light and darkness that generates the physical universe and it is *Oya* who keeps this interaction in a constant state of flux and motion.

There is no literal translation for the word *Ifá*; it refers to a religious tradition, an understanding of ethics, a process of spiritual transformation and a set of scriptures that are the basis for a complex system of divination.

Ifá is found throughout the African diaspora where it spread as an integral part of Yoruba culture. The Yoruba Nation is located in the Southwestern region of Nigeria. Prior to colonization, the Yoruba Nation was a federation of city-states that was originally centered in the city of *Ilẹ́ Ifẹ*. According to *Ifá* myth, the Yorubas migrated to *Ilẹ́ Ifẹ* from the East under the leadership of a warrior chief named *Oduduwa*. It is difficult to date the time of the Yoruba move into West Africa because of limited archaeological research on the subject. Estimates range from between sixteen hundred to twenty-five hundred years ago. It is likely that migration took place over a number of generations. As the population grew, each new city-state that became a part of the Yoruba federation was governed by a chief called "*Oba*". The position of *Oba* is a form of hereditary monarchy and each *Oba* goes through an initiation that makes them a spiritual descendant of *Oduduwa*.

Traditional Yoruba political institutions are very much integrated with traditional Yoruba religious institutions. Both structures survived British rule in Nigeria, and continue to function alongside the current civil government.

Within the discipline of *Ifá*, there is a body of wisdom called "*awo*", which attempts to preserve the rituals that create direct communication with Forces in Nature. *Awo* is a Yoruba word that is usually translated to mean "secret". Unfortunately, there is no real English equivalent to the word *awo*, because the word carries strong cultural and esoteric associations. In traditional Yoruba culture. *awo* refers to the hidden principles that explain the Mystery of Creation and Evolution. *Awo* is the esoteric understanding of the invisible forces that sustain dynamics and form within Nature. The essence of these invisible forces is not considered secret because they are devious, they are secret because they remain elusive, awesome in their power to transform and not readily apparent. As such they can only be grasped through direct interaction and participation. Anything which can be known by the intellect alone ceases to be *awo*.

The primal inspiration for *awo* is the communication between transcendent Spiritual Forces and human consciousness. This communication is believed to be facilitated by the Spirit of *Eṣu*, who is the Divine Messenger. Working in close association with *Eṣu* is *Ogun*, who is the Spirit of Iron. *Ogun* has the power to clear away those obstacles that stand in the way of spiritual growth. According to *Ifá*, the work done by *Ogun* is guided by *Ochosi*, who as the Spirit of the Tracker has the ability to locate the shortest path to our spiritual goals. The essential goal that *Ochosi* is called upon to guide us towards is the task of building "*ìwa-pèlé*", which means "good character". This guidance takes the form of a spiritual quest which is called "*ìwakiri*". One of the functions of *Obatala* is to preserve the Mystic Vision that to those who make the quest of *ìwakiri* in search of *ìwa-pèlé*.

The power of *Oya* is described by *Ifá* as one of many Spiritual Forces in Nature which are called "*Orisha*". The word *Orisha* means "Select Head". In a cultural context, *Orisha* is a reference to the various Forces in Nature that guide consciousness. According to *Ifá*, everything in Nature has some form of consciousness called "*Orí*". The *Orí* of all animals, plants and humans is believed to be guided by a specific Force in Nature (*Orisha*) which defines the quality of a particular form of consciousness. There are a large number of *Orisha* and each *Orisha* has its own *awo*.

The unique function of *Oya* within the realm of *Orisha Awo* (Mysteries of Nature) is to provide the those changing conditions that force consciousness to grow, expand and transcend its limitations. To call an *Orisha* the Spirit of the Wind is to make a symbolic reference to constant motion that exists in Nature. The reference to Wind is not limited to the wind that blows across the surface of the Earth. Wind is a phenomena that occurs throughout Creation causing shifts and movement throughout all that exists. If it were not for the random element of change as represented by Oya, everything that existed in the Universe would have the same texture, structure and appearance.

Ifá teaches that all Forces in Nature come into Being through the manifestation of energy patterns called *Odu*. *Ifá* has identified and labeled 256 different *Odu* which can be thought of as different expressions of consciousness. But because consciousness itself is generated by *Obatala* every *Odu* contains an element of *Obatala's* *aşę* (power).

In metaphysical terms, this means that all of Creation is linked to *Obatala* as the Source of Being. *Ifá* teaches that all forms of consciousness contain a spark of *aşę* (spiritual power) from *Obatala*, and it is this spark that links everything that is to its shared Beginning. It is *Oya* who has the task of shaking the divergent aspects of consciousness in such a way that consciousness continues to evolve. *Oya* is the Force in Nature that insures that there is no stagnation in any corner of Creation.

In addition, *Oya* supplies the gateway that links cycles of *atunwa* (reincarnation). *Ifá* teaches that persons come back to life on Earth through the process of rebirth. Every individual has a soul called "*emí*", which survives physical death and dwells in *Ikolę Ǫrun*, which is the invisible Realm of the Ancestors. While the *emí* is in *Ikolę Ǫrun* it is capable of making contact with those who live on earth. This contact is facilitated through the

Spiritual Winds that link the Realm of the Ancestors with Earth.
This Wind is at the heart of *Oya's* power and makes *Oya* an
essential participant in those ceremonies which honor the memory
of the Ancestors.

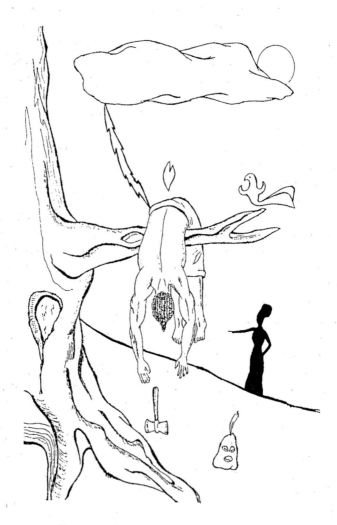

Oya invoking the elevation of Shango

I.

ALỌ IRINTÀN OYA
FOLKTALES OF THE SPIRIT OF THE WIND

A. *OYA KO SÍ 'KU* — The Spirit of the Wind Protects Us From Death

It was *Oya* (Spirit of the Wind) who advised *Ọrúnmìlà* to cast *Ifá* on the day that *Iku* (the Spirit of Death) was planning to journey past his home. *Ọrúnmìlà* heeded the warning and placed a plate of yams, a bowl of soup and a cooked chicken on the refuse heap near his home.

As *Iku* (the Spirit of Death) approached the house he saw the food on the refuse heap and sat down to eat. When he had finished his meal he spotted *Ọrúnmìlà* and gave chase. The food slowed him down and *Iku* was unable to catch his intended prey.

Speaking to him from a distance, *Ọrúnmìlà* asked *Iku* why he had come to *Ikolẹ Ayẹ* (Earth). *Iku* said "I have come to fetch someone who was thoughtless. I was to take him with me to the land of the ancestors. But I cannot be rude to someone who has offered me a meal."

Commentary: The *Ifá* concept of Destiny includes the belief that every person has a pre-ordained time of passing. This time cannot be extended, but it can be shortened. Those who do not live their life to the full time allowed are considered careless in their efforts to live in harmony with self and world.

Ọrúnmìlà was able to avert his premature death by making the proper offerings to *Iku* at a time when death was near. In the story it was *Oya* who warned *Ọrúnmìlà* of the presence of death. *Ifá* cosmology closely associates *Oya* with a Spiritual Force called *Ajalaiye*. The *Ajalaiye* are hot winds that blow close to the earth. These winds play a positive role in the process of replenishing the soil, but they also carry the kind of germs that cause epidemics in West Africa.

Orúnmìlà was able to avoid *Iku* because he was sensitive to the message from the Spirit of the Wind.

B. *OYA 'YA SHANGO* — The Spirit of the Wind as Wife of the Spirit of Lightning

Shango (The Spirit of Lightning) was the fourth *Alafin* (Regional Chief) of *Oyo*. It was a time when the Yoruba Nation was plagued by war and internal conflict. In an effort to bring stability to the Nation, *Shango* united the kingdom of *Oyo*. When the days of battle and strife came to an end, *Shango* sat in his palace and suffered from boredom. In an effort to recreate the excitement of his youth, he ordered his brothers, *Timi* and *Gbonkaa* to fight a duel.

Timi and *Gbonkaa* came to the compound of the *Alafin* (Regional Chief) and played their *bata* (sacred drums) until *Timi* fell asleep and *Gbonkaa* declared himself the winner. *Shango* was not satisfied and ordered them to return to fight again.

Timi and *Gbonkaa* came to the compound of the *Alafin* (Regional Chief) on the following day prepared for battle. *Timi* strung his bow and began hurling arrows at *Gbonkaa*. None of the arrows hit their target because *Gbonkaa* was wearing the *ogun* (medicine) of protection. *Gbonkaa* repeated the incantations that put *Timi* asleep, then stood over his body and cut off his head.

When the people of *Oyo* saw *Timi* dead at the palace they became angry at *Shango* and drove him from the compound. Overcome with grief, *Shango* left the city of *Oyo* and hung himself. The first person to find his body was his wife *Oya* who said, "*Oba ko so*" which means, "The Chief is not dead."

Commentary: The Myth of *Shango* is based upon a historical figure who created a federation of city-states along the Eastern rim of the Yoruba Nation. The region had been plagued by internal wars, which made it vulnerable to slave traders from the regions North of the rain forest.

This Myth has several variations which put a slightly different emphasis on the role of *Shango* in relationship to the brothers *Timi* and *Gbonkaa*. In some versions, *Timi* and *Gbonkaa* are involved in political intrigue. *Shango* becomes angry at their actions and unleashes his aggression in an excessive way, causing the deaths of many innocent people in the city of *Oyo*. The more common version of the myth has *Shango* pitting the two brothers against each other for his own amusement and out of jealousy for their popularity among the people of *Oyo*.

In both versions, *Shango* is accused of committing an offense which makes him unworthy to serve as the *Alafin*. Yoruba culture is based on hereditary Patriarchal chieftaincies. The conduct of a political chief is monitored by a council of male and female elders called "*Ogboni*". If the council of elders believes that the chief has flagrantly abused the power of his position they can insist that the chief be removed from office. In pre-colonial times the chief could not simply step down from his position. If he was removed from office he was expected to commit suicide. This was usually done by ingesting poison, which he would drink as part of a rite of passage that would prepare him for entry into the realm of the ancestors.

Most of the versions of the *Shango* Myth have him take his own life by hanging from a tree. In some versions of the Myth it is an *iroko* tree and in others the tree is the *ayan* tree. Both trees are sacred to the ancestors and are used as communal shrines in places where these trees are located near a town. This portion of the Myth suggests that *Shango* realizes his mistake before he comes under censor by *Ogboni* and attempts to avoid the shame and guilt of censor by the elders by taking his own life.

The appearance of *Oya* at the moment of the hanging insures that *Shango's* spirit will become transformed as he passes into the realm of the ancestors. This Myth is the *Ifá* expression of the dynamics of death and resurrection. Because of the belief in reincarnation the resurrection is not the physical reappearance of *Shango* in physical form. It is the elevation of the *emi*, or soul of

Shango to a place where it returns to source and becomes merged with the power of lightning.

This identification may seem confusing to those who are used to the Western concept of linear time. The Myth of *Shango* is rooted in the *Ifá* concept of circular time. According to *Ifá* the process of spiritual transformation is both preparation for future cycles of reincarnation and a return to the primal source of consciousness. By realizing his mistake, *Shango* prepares for his next life and becomes reunited by the spirit of fire which gave birth to his own personal consciousness. The presence of *Oya* serves to open those passageways that allow this identification to take place.

This story established the scriptural basis for *Oya's* sacred function within *Ẹgbẹ́ Egúngun* (Ancestral Reverence Societies). It is the female initiates of *Oya* who frequently have the task of invoking possession in the male mediums who wear the colored cloth of *Egúngun* ritual. *Oya* as the Spirit of the Wind has the power to open the gateways between *Ikolẹ Ọrun* (The Invisible Realm of the Ancestors) and *Ikolẹ Ayẹ* (Earth). This pathway is opened through the use of *"Ajalaiyẹ"*, which means "Winds of Earth", and *"Ajalọrun"*, which means "Winds of the Ancestral Realm". It is these Spirit Winds that are used as roadways between the human dimension and the ancestral dimension. This Wind should not be confused with the winds that effect weather on the planet. They are lines of *aṣẹ* (power) which exist in the invisible atmosphere that links the Spiritual World with the Physical World.

In metaphysical terms the relationship between *Oya* and *Shango* is one of eternal polarity. *Shango* is the lightning that is generated by the wind. *Shango* gains his potency through the *aṣẹ* (power) that is generated by *Oya*. *Ifá* teaches that all *aṣẹ* (power) is generated by the relationship between forces of expansion and forces of contraction. In *Ifá* scripture forces of expansion are usually characterized as male *Orisha* and forces of contraction are usually characterized as female *Orisha*. It is the force of the wind that contracts in a circular movement that generates the static electricity that bursts from the sky after the current is concentrated in a small area. This is a literal manifestation of the interaction between male and female principles of power as they exist in Nature.

C. *OYA GALÀ'BINRIN* — The Spirit of the Wind as Deer Woman

Oya made the journey from *Ikolę Qrun* (The Realm of the Ancestors) to *Ikolę Ayę* (Earth) in the form of an antelope on the day that she wanted to sell her goods in the market. Every five days *Oya* was able to change her shape from *galà* (deer) to *obinrin* (woman). *Oya* waited five days, then entered the market carrying a bundle of multicolored cloth. It was on that day that *Shango* (Spirit of Lightning) became overwhelmed by her beauty.

Oya ignored *Shango's* efforts to make her acquaintance. Instead, she sold her cloth, left the market and headed into the forest. Because he was struck by her beauty, *Shango* followed *Oya* into the forest, where he watched her put on the skin of *galà* (deer) and transformed herself into a creature of the jungle.

Five days later *Shango* returned to the same place and watched *Oya* transform herself back into a woman. As she headed for the market, *Shango* took her animal skin and placed it in his sack. Later that day *Oya* returned to the forest and made a desperate search for her skin. Because *Oya* could not live in the bush without her animal skin she agreed to return with *Shango* to his home and become his wife.

Shango had two senior wives; *Oshun* (The Spirit of the *Oshun* River) and *Oba* (The Spirit of the *Oba* River). In time *Oshun* and *Oba* became jealous of the favored treatment that *Oya* received from *Shango*. *Oshun* and *Oba* told *Oya* that they thought she was crude, and that she behaved like an animal. Because *Oya* did not want the women to discover her secret, she renewed her search for her skin. When she found the skin in *Shango's* sack, she took it and returned to the forest.

Shango felt grief when he found that *Oya* had left him. He followed her into the forest until he spotted a *galà* (deer) with two powerful horns. The beast was digging a hoof into the dirt and had its head lowered in preparation for battle. It was on that day that

Shango recognized the *galà* as *Oya*. Instead of lifting his bow, *Shango* offered the animal a plate of *akara* (bean cakes). *Oya* removed the horns from her head and presented them to *Shango* in return for his kindness.

From that day on *Shango* has used the horns of the *galà* to call the Spirit of *Oya*.

Commentary: *Ifá* teaches that *Orisha* exist at all levels of Being. This means that the Spirit of the Wind can be found in the gas storms that swirl around exploded stars, *Oya* can be found in the Wind that blows across the surface of the Earth, and *Oya* appears in the animal realm as a horned deer.

Ifá also teaches that all things evolve from a single source and that all things are interconnected and interrelated. This means that the process of becoming attuned to *Awo 'ya* (The Mystery of the Spirit of the Wind) involves a sense of empathy and deep spiritual bonding with many different dimensions of reality.

In this story *Oya* shifts between manifestation as human and animal. The point of the story is that all things within the Universe have consciousness and deserve respect. Each of us is linked psychically and biologically to all the life forms that have evolved into human nature.

Ifá also teaches that it is possible to learn lessons from Nature through mystical identification with certain animal forms. In this instance it is the deer who teaches the lesson of tolerance, acceptance and compassion.

Oya is often described as a warrior, which is accurate. However, her *aşę* as a warrior comes through her ability to invoke the assistance of elemental spirits such as deer and birds to assist her in battle. This ability gives *Oya* a key role in the protection of those who are going through the process of initiation. It also makes *Oya* one of the guardians of issues related to the fair treatment of women.

II.

ÌM̀Ọ̀ OYA
THE THEOLOGICAL FUNCTION OF THE
SPIRIT OF THE WIND

A. OYA 'YÀNMỌ́-ÌPIN — The Spirit of the Wind and the Concept of Destiny

The *Ifá* concept of *"àyànmọ́-ìpin"*, which means "Destiny", is based on the belief that each person chooses their individual destiny before being born into the world. These choices materialize as those components that form human potential. Within the scope of each person's potential there exists parameters of choice that can enhance or inhibit the fullest expression of individual destiny. *Ifá* calls these possibilities *"ọ̀na ipin"*, which means "road of destiny". Each decision that is made in the course of one lifetime can effect the range of possibilities that exists in the future, by either limiting or expanding the options for growth.

It is within the context of choice, or what is known in Western philosophical tradition as "free will" that *Ifá* recognizes a collection of Spiritual Forces called *"Ibora"*. In Yoruba, the word *Ibora* means "Warrior". Traditionally the *Ibora* include *Eṣu*, *Ògún* and *Ochosi*. *Eṣu* is the cornerstone that links the *Ibora* as they relate to the issue of spiritual growth. According to *Ifá*, each moment of existence includes a wide range of possible actions, reactions and interpretations. Those moments which require decisive action are described in *Ifá* scripture as *"ọ̀na'pade"*, which means "junction in the road". Whenever a person who is trying to build character through the use of *Ifá* spiritual discipline reaches *ọ̀na'pade*, it is customary to consult *Eṣu* regarding the question of which path will bring blessings from *Orisha*.

Ifá teaches that blessings come to those who make choices that are consistent with their highest destiny. Within Yoruba culture it is understood that an individual's highest destiny is based on those choices that build "*ìwa-pèlé*", which means "good character". Those who develop good character are often described as weaving white cloth, which means creating purity and spiritual elevation in the world. The collective impact of those who weave white cloth is entering into a state of mystical union with the Chief, or the Source of White Cloth who is called "*Obatala*". This is true for everyone, even those who worship other *Orisha*. *Ifá* scripture clearly suggests what all of the *Orisha* exist as an extension of the power of consciousness that is created by the *aṣẹ* (power) of *Obatala*.

The relationship between *Oya* and *Obatala* has several dimensions. As the guardian of the gateway to the Realm of the Ancestors, *Oya* has a ceremonial role in the preservation of the wisdom of the ancestors. *Ifá* ancestor reverence is based on the belief that we become who we are by standing on the shoulders of those who have gone before us. Those who are initiated into *Awo Oya* (Mysteries of the Spirit of the Wind) have the keys for unlocking the wisdom of the past as a constant source of inspiration and guidance. *Obatala* is the guardian of *ìwa-pèlé* (good character), and it is *Oya* who brings the voice of those ancestors who preserved the wisdom that leads to the development of good character.

Oya also has the role of disrupting complacency. *Ifá* teaches that the process of seeking harmony and balance with self and world is an ongoing process which requires constant attention, vigilance and wisdom. It is possible to live under the illusion that your life is in harmony with its own destiny and in harmony with Forces in Nature that exist in the world. *Ifá* scripture suggests that when a person is in a state of illusion they will eventually run up against those Forces in Nature that will shatter the illusion. *Oya* is one of those Forces. The Wind as a Spiritual Principle brings the unexpected, the chaotic, the transformative and the overwhelming Forces of Nature that give human consciousness a sense of mortality and humility.

B. *OYA ONITOJU AȘẸ* — The Spirit of the Source of Change

Ifá cosmology is based on the belief that the Primal Source of Creation is a form of Spiritual Essence called "*aşẹ*". There is no literal translation for *aşẹ*, although it is used in prayer to mean "May it be so".

Ifá teaches that the visible universe is generated by two dynamic forces. One is the force of "*inàlo*", which means "expansion", and the other is the force of "*isoki*", which means "contraction". The first initial manifestation of these forces is through "*imò*", which means "light", and through "*aimoyẹ*", which means "darkness". In *Ifá* myth expansion and light are frequently identified with Male Spirits called "*Orisha'ko*". Contraction and darkness are frequently identified with Female Spirits called "*Orisha'bo*". Neither manifestation of *aşẹ* is considered superior to the other and both are viewed as essential elements in the overall balance of Nature.

In *Ifá* cosmology both *imò* and *aimoyẹ* arise from the matrix of the invisible universe which is called "*Imolẹ*", which means "House of Light". Within the house of light there is an invisible substance that transforms spiritual potential into physical reality. The invisible substance that moves between these two dimensions is called *aşẹ*, and it is *Obatala* who brings the *aşẹ* of Light into the world. If there was nothing but light in the world, the universe would burn, then fade.

It is the constant interaction between light and dark, between expansion and contraction, between fusion and fission that gives shape to the universe. If these polarities always interacted in the same way, the universe would be made up of stars that were all the same size, planets that were all the same shape, land would be similar all over the Earth and everyone would look the same. One of the most perplexing aspects of Creation to Western science is the fact that there exists a wide range of variation within every aspect of Being. Western science call this the result of chaos; *Ifá* says that it is the result of the *aṣẹ* of *Oya*.

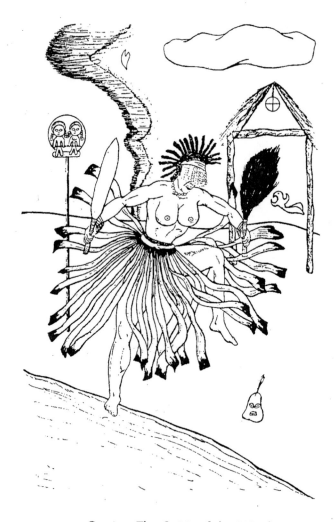

Oya — The Spirit of the Wind

III.

ÒNA OYA
THE ROADS OF THE SPIRIT OF THE WIND

The word *Oya* is an elision of the *Oriki* (Praise Name) *Omo Iyan sa*, which means, "Child of the Mother of Nine". In the West, *Yansa* is used as a synonym for *Oya*. However, the *Oriki* suggests that *Oya* is the child of *Yansa* and that *Yansa* is the Mother of the Spirit of the Wind. Two aspects of *Oya* which make frequent appearance in *Ifá* scripture are "*Ajalaiyẹ*" which means "Winds of the Earth", and "*Ajalọrun*", which means "Winds of the Realm of the Ancestors".

IV.

ILẸ́ ORISHA
THE SHRINE OF THE SPIRIT OF THE WIND

A. *ILẸ́ ORISHA ADURA* — Shrine for Prayer and Meditation to the Spirit of the Wind

Those who are interested in honoring *Oya* who have no access to either *Ifá* or *Orisha* elders can set up a shrine that may be used for meditation and prayer. The shrine can be used as a focal point for meditation that can lead to a deeper awareness, appreciation and understanding of *Oya's* role and function within Nature. Such a shrine should be set up in a clean place and make use of multicolored cloth as a setting for other symbolic altar pieces. Pictures of powerful and disruptive Forces in Nature such as volcanoes, hurricanes, tornadoes and thunderstorms would reflect the quality of *Oya's* inner nature.

Oya is also associated with bush cow and seven spiritual manifestations of birds. The birds are used in association with the female mysteries of *"Iyami"*, which means "My Mothers". These spirit birds are used to induce astral travel, clairvoyance, and provide healing to those who suffer from otherwise incurable illness.

B. *ILẸ́ ORISHA ORIKI* — Shrine for Invocation to the Spirit of the Wind

Shrines which are used for the invocation of *Oya* are constructed from consecrated religious elements that are presented to a devotee during initiation. These objects may vary, but they generally include a pot that contains the sacred power objects that attract the *aṣẹ* (spiritual essence) of *Oya*, a rattle made from seed in a pod, a black horse tail fan, a *sekere* (beaded rattle), and weapons made from copper.

The *Ifá* calender is based on a five day week and those who have received the *aṣẹ* of *Orisha* generally greet their shrine each morning and say invocations to their shrine every five days. The invocations are called "*Oriki*", which means "praising the con-sciousness". An example of *Oriki Oya* is as follows:

> ***Iba ṣẹ Oya Oluweku.***
>> I respect the Spirit of the Wind, Chief of the Ances-tors.
>
> ***Iba ṣẹ Opere Lalaoyan.***
>> I respect She Who Walks with Confidence and Pride.
>
> ***Iba ṣẹ Oya yeba Iya mesa Oyo.***
>> I respect the Spirit of the Wind, the Senior Mother of Oyo.
>
> ***Ajalaiyẹ afẹfẹ Iku lẹlẹ bioke.***
>> The Winds of Earth carry the Ancestors.
>
> ***Ajalọrun afẹfẹ iku lele biokẹ.***
>> The Winds of the Invisible Realm carry the Ancestors.
>
> ***Ajalaiyẹ, Ajalọrun fun mi ni 're.***
>> May the Winds of Earth and the Winds of the Invisible Realm bring me good fortune.
>
> ***Oya winiwini.***
>> The Spirit of the Wind is wondrous.
>
> ***Iba se Oya l'o ni Egún.***
>> I respect the Spirit of the Wind who Guides the Ancestors.
>
> ***Iya mi oro bi omu sẹ l'aiya.***
>> Mother fill me with the wisdom of your breasts.
>
> ***Iba ṣẹ Omo Yansan.***
>> I respect the child of the Mother of Nine.
>
> ***Mbẹ mbẹ Yansan.***
>> May the Mother of Nine exist forever.
>
> ***Aṣẹ.***
>> May it be so.

C. *ADIMU OYA* — Offerings to the Spirit of the Wind

In all forms of *Ifá* and *Orisha* worship it is traditional to make an offering whenever guidance or assistance is requested from Spiritual Forces. *Adimu* is a term that is generally used to refer to food and drink that is presented to the Spirit of a particular shrine. The idea behind the process of making an offering is that it would be unfair to ask for something for nothing. Those who have an unconsecrated shrine to *Oya* can make the offering in their own words. Those who have a consecrated shrine to *Oya* may use the *Oriki* for *Oya* when making a presentation of *Adimu*. This is usually done when a prayer requesting assistance from *Oya* is made. The answer to the prayer can then come through divination.

The traditional forms of *adimu* offered if *Oya* include:

1. Eggplant
2. Red wine

D. *EBO OYA* — Life Force Offerings to the Spirit of the Wind

There is a wide range of ritual procedure in Africa involving the worship of *Orisha*. Many of the differences in ceremonial process reflect regional differences in emphasis rather than essence. The term, "life force offering" is used in reference to the fact that many *Orisha* rituals require a preparation of a feast or communal meal. Whenever this occurs the blood from the animal that is used for the meal is given to *Orisha* as an offering. This offering is considered a reaffirmation between *Ikolę Ǫrun* (The Realm of the Ancestors) and *Ikolę Ayę* (Earth). This covenant is an agreement between Spirit and humans that Spirit will provide food for the nourishment of people on earth. In return, the worshipers of *Ifá* and *Orisha* agree to respect the spirit of the animal who provided the food and agree to elevate the spirit of that animal so it will return to provide food for future generations.

Whenever a life force offering is made to any of the *Orisha*, an invocation is generally made to *Ogun* as part of the process. This is a grossly misunderstood aspect of *Ifá* and *Orisha* worship which has suffered from negative stereotypes in the press and the media. It is part of *awo Ogun* (Mystery of the Spirit of Iron) to learn the inner secrets of making life force offerings. When an *Orisha* initiate is making a life force offering it should include an invocation for the *Odu Ogunda*. If the initiate is using the *Lucumí* system of *Merindinlogun*, the invocation would be to *Ogunda Meji*. In *Ifá* the invocation for life force offerings is to *Ogunda-Irętę*.

The traditional life force offerings fro *Oya* include:

1. Hen
2. Ram
3. Sheep
4. Goat

E. *ÌWȨ OYA* — Cleansing for the Spirit of the Wind

Ifá and *Orisha* makes extensive use of a wide range of cleansing rituals that are designed to clear away the negative effects of illness, sorrow, grief, anger and contamination by negative spiritual influences. The most fundamental form of cleansings takes the form of blessing water. This means that the water is charged with the power of prayer to accomplish a specific purpose. Once the water has been blessed it can be used to wash specific parts of the body such as the head, the hands or the feet, or it can be used for bathing.

Those who are uninitiated may say a prayer to *Oya* in their own language and breathe the prayer into the water. It is also common for *Oya* to make use of a broom for cleansing work. The following prayer may be used for both water and the broom by those who have been initiated in *Awo 'ya* (Mysteries of the Spirit of the Wind).

Those who are initiated may add their *aşę* to the water with the following prayer:

Iba ṣẹ Oya gbe nla ijo mora.
> I respect the Spirit of the Wind who dances with big movements.

Oya b'a mi de 'di a agbo omo mi.
> Spirit of the Wind, touch my child's medicine.

K'o mu, ko ki.
> Make it strong and powerful.

Kieso omo mi di pupo gun rẹrẹ.
> Let my child be blessed for the good.

Ajalaiyẹ Ajalọrun mo be yin,
> I beg the Winds of Earth and the Winds of the Invisible Realm,

Mimi r'owo san awin Ọrun mi ati beebee.
> May I always do good things in the World.

Aṣẹ.
> May it be so.

Following the cleansing, empty the water somewhere away from the entrance to your home. If a broom is being used clean the broom by rubbing it in the Earth.

F. *OYA IYA 'JA* — The Spirit of the Wind, Mother of the Market Place

In rural regions of Nigeria most Yoruba cities are founded on a farming economy. The cities are surrounded by communal farms that are generally run by specific extended families. Traditionally the men work on the farms and the women sell the excess produce in the market. Rural markets are usually located in the center of town, are open air and are consecrated to *Oya*. There is frequently an altar to *Oya* at either the center or the gateway to the market. The altar varies from a simple mound of dirt to elaborate shrines. Once a year offerings are brought to the market place at the market festival.

Because of her association with commerce, *Oya* is frequently called upon as a source of abundance. It is common for women in Nigeria to bring a handful of cornmeal to the market place, pray

on the grain, then toss it near the entrance to the market. For those
who have a consecrated shrine to *Oya* the following prayer may
be used:

>*Ire ni mo nwa l'owo o to.*
>>It is abundance that I am searching for.
>
>*Oya re'le Egúngun lo lo're wa fun mi owo ni nwa l'owo mi o to.*
>>Spirit of the Wind, go to the house of the Ancestors and bring me abundance.
>
>*Oya gbe rẹrẹ ko ni Olu-gbe-rẹrẹ.*
>>Spirit of the Wind bring me good things from the Chief of Good things.
>
>*Bi ojo ba la maa la.*
>>When the day breaks abundance will come to me.
>
>*A dupẹ.*
>>I give thanks.
>
>*Aṣẹ.*
>>May it be so.

V.

ORISHA 'GUN
THE SPIRIT OF THE WIND AND THE MEANING OF SPIRIT POSSESSION

Those who practice the religion of *Ifá* in Africa are generally members of a society that worships a single *Orisha*. These societies are usually referred to by the term "*ẹ̀gbẹ́*", which means "heart", as in the expression "the heart of the matter". Those who worship *Oya* would be members of *Ẹ̀gbẹ́ Oya*. There are regional differences in the use of this term. In some areas societies of *Oya* worship might be called either "*Ilẹ́ Oya*", meaning "House of *Oya*", or "*Awon Oya*", meaning, "Those who worship *Oya*".

Regardless of the name used, each of these societies preserves the oral history, myth and wisdom associated with *Awo Oya* (The Mystery of the Wind). Part of the wisdom that is preserved concerns the discipline used to access altered states of consciousness. Western literature on *Orisha* tends to refer to these states as "possession". This term is inadequate to describe the various forms of trance that are used to assist the *Orisha* worshiper in their understanding of the Mysteries of Being.

Ifá teaches that it is possible to access both *Orisha* (Forces in Nature) and *Egun* (ancestors) through the disciplined use of dreams. The word "*àlá*" is used in Yoruba to mean "dream". *Ala* is the last part of the word *Obatala* and it suggests that the dream state is closely associated with the source of consciousness itself. The word "*alála*" is the word for "dreamer". Because dreamer has a positive connotation in *Ifá*, the word *alála* is a reference to those who are able to make effective use of dreams. *Alala* appears to be a contraction of *ala* and *ala*. In Yoruba words are often repeated for emphasis or to establish relative relationships. To use the word `alá twice suggests that the reference to dreamer is an expression of the belief that dreams can access the true source of inner thoughts.

Ifá teaches that it is possible to develop an ongoing relationship with *Orisha* that makes a person sensitive to the influence of *Orisha* on a daily basis that effects their immediate environment. In English this is usually referred to as a highly developed intuition. The Yoruba word for intuition is "*ogbon inu*", which translates literally to mean "the stomach of the earth". *Ifá* metaphysics is based on the idea that those Forces in Nature that sustain life on earth establish certain guidelines for living in harmony with Creation. The development of a sensitivity to these forces is part of the discipline of *Orisha* worship and this sensitivity is called "*ogbon inu*".

There are a number of words that are used to describe those altered states that are commonly referred to as possession. In conjunction with *Orisha* the word "*jogun*", meaning either "I possess" or "I have", is used to describe a close spiritual connection with Spirit. The phrase "*Orisha'gun*", is used to describe those who have assumed the characteristics of a particular *Orisha*.

The more common term for possession is "*ini*". This word reveals the *Ifá* perspective on those trance states which represent a deep connection with the *aşę* (power) of *Orisha*. The word *ini* appears to be a contraction of "*i*", which is a personal pronoun, and "*ni*", which is the verb "to be". To use the phrase "I am" as a reference to possession suggests that what is frequently thought of as an intrusion from outside forces is more accurately understood as a process of unlocking the *awo* (mystery) of the inner self. *Ifá* teaches that every person comes to Earth with a spark of divinity at the foundation of their *ori* (inner spirit). Part of the discipline of *Orisha* worship is to access this spark of divinity. This is generally accomplished through initiation, which is designed to guide the initiate towards access to the inner self, which in turn forms a transcendent link to that *Orisha* which is closest to the consciousness of the initiate.

Those who have been through initiation for *Oya* can enhance their access to *ini* at the same time that offerings are made to their shrine on a five day cycle. This is done by saying *Oriki Oya* in front of the initiate's *Oya* shrine. When the *Oriki* is spoken a candle is lit near the *Orisha* pot and a glass of water is placed near the candle. After the *Oriki* has been completed, the initiate breathes into the glass of water and says the word "*to*", which means "enough". The word *to* is used at the end of *Oriki* as a seal or lock to attach the invocation to whatever it is spoken onto.

Using the index finger, the ring finger and the little finger on the left hand, the initiate dips the fingers in the water and runs the water from between the forehead across the top of the head and down the back of the neck. When the fingers are between the eyebrows say, "*iwaju*", which is the name of the power center at the forehead. When the fingers are on the top of the head say, "*ori*" which is the name of the power center at the crown of the skull. When the fingers are on the back of the neck say, "*ipako*", which is the name of the power center at the base of the skull.

A sample of the type of *Oriki* that is used for this process is as follows:

> *Iba şę Oya o rin n'eru ojikutu s'eru.*
>> I respect the Spirit of the Wind who does not fear death.
>
> *Iyagba n'lę Ifon alabalaşę oba patapa n'ilę iranję.*
>> Mother of the Realm of the Ancestors is the one who guides all future generations.
>
> *Oya, gbę nla ijo mora.*
>> Spirit of the Wind who dances with big movements.
>
> *Oya o pę o.*
>> Spirit of the Wind I am calling you.
>
> *Oya o pę o.*
>> Spirit of the Wind I am calling you.
>
> *Oya o pę o.*
>> Spirit of the Wind I am calling you.
>
> *Oya o pę o.*
>> Spirit of the Wind I am calling you.

Oya ro.
   Spirit of the Wind descend.
Efufu lẹlẹ ti nda igi lokelokẹ,
   Strong Wind that clears a path,
A dupẹ̀.
   I thank you.
Aṣẹ.
   May it be so.

VI.

ORIN OYA
SONG FOR THE SPIRIT OF THE WIND

Call: *E i ekua e i ekua Oya sile kunfoyawo awode ara koyumariwo*
        Oyade.
        (The dead, the dead, In the house of the Spirit of the Wind
        She wears the palm fronds of the Spirit of the Wind).
Response: Repeat.
Call: *Ara koyumariwo.*
        (She wears the palm fronds)
Response: *Oyadę.*
        (Spirit of the Wind arise)
Call: *Ara koyumaiwo.*
        (She wears the palm fronds)
Response: *Oyadę.*
        (Spirit of the Wind arise)
Call: *Agogo Oya agogo Oya agogo ito ito Oya.*
        (Greetings to the Spirit of the Wind)
Response: Repeat.
Call *Oya il' Oya.*
        (The Spirit of the Wind, the House of the Spirit of the Wind)

Call: *Oya winiwini Oya winiwini.*
        (Spirit of the Wind exist forever, Spirit of the Wind exist
        forever)
Response: *Oyansa Oya winiwini.*
        (Mother of Nine, Spirit of the Wind exist forever)
Call: *Oya winiwini Oya winiwini.*
        (Spirit of the Wind exist forever, Spirit of the Wind exist
        forever)

Response: ***Oyansa Oya winiwini.***
    (Mother of Nine, Spirit of the Wind exist forever)
Call: ***Yansa winiwini Oya winiwini.***
    (Mother of Nine exist forever, Spirit of the Wind exist forever)
Response: ***Oyansa Oya winiwini.***
    (Mother of Nine, Spirit of the Wind exist forever)

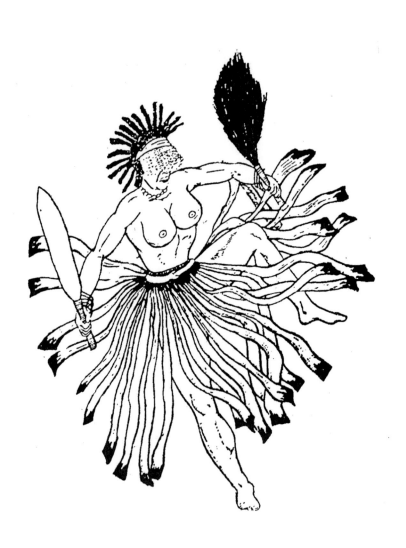

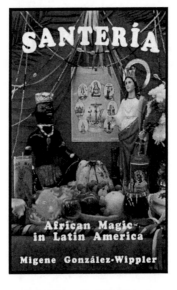

SANTERIA

AFRICAN MAGIC
IN LATIN AMERICA

BY MIGENE GONZALEZ WIPPLER

In 1973, the first hardcover edition of *Santeria: African Magic in Latin America* by cultural anthropologist Migene Gonzalez-Wippler was first published by Julian Press. It became an immediate best-seller and is still considered by many experts one of the most popular books on Santeria, having gone through 4 editions and several translations. Now this beloved classic, written by one the foremost scholars on the Afro-Cuban religion, has returned in a 5th edition. This time the text has been carefully edited and corrected to incorporate vital new material. The beliefs, practices, legends of Santeria are brilliantly brought to life in this exciting and critically acclaimed best-seller. If you ever wondered what Santeria is, if you are curious about the rituals and practices of this mysterious religion, and want to delve in its deepest secrets, this book will answer all your questions and much more.

ISBN 0-942272-04-8 5½"x 8½" $14.95

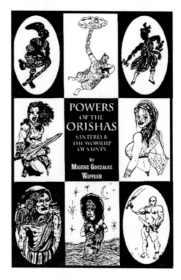

POWERS OF THE ORISHAS
Santeria and the Worship of Saints
Migene Gonzalez Wippler

Santeria is the Afro-Cuban religion based on an amalgamation between some of the magio-religious beliefs and practices of the Yoruba people and those of the Catholic church. In Cuba where the Yoruba proliferated extensively, they became known as *Lucumi,* a word that means "friendship".

Santeria is known in Cuba as Lucumi Religion. The original Yoruba language, interspersed with Spanish terms and corrupted through the centuries of misuse and mispronunciation, also became known as Lucumi. Today some of the terms used in Santeria would not be recognized as Yoruba in Southwestern Nigeria, the country of origin of the Yoruba people.

Santeria is a Spanish term that means a confluence of saints and their worship. These saints are in reality clever disguises for some of the Yoruba deities, known as Orishas. During the slave trade, the Yoruba who were brought to Cuba were forbidden the practice of their religion by their Spanish masters. In order to continue their magical and religious observances safely the slaves opted for the identification and disguise of the Orishas with some of the Catholic saints worshipped by the Spaniards. In this manner they were able to worship their deities under the very noses of the Spaniards without danger of punishment.

Throughout the centuries the practices of the Yoruba became very popular and soon many other people of the Americas began to practice the new religion.

ISBN 0-942272-25-0 5½"x 8½" 144 pages $9.95

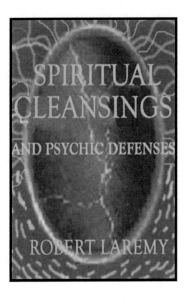

$9.95

SPIRITUAL CLEANSINGS & PSYCHIC DEFENSES

By Robert Laremy

Psychic attacks are real and their effects can be devastating to the victim. Negative vibrations can be as harmful as bacteria, germs and viruses. There are time-honored methods of fighting these insidious and pernicious agents of distress. These techniques are described in this book and they can be applied by you. No special training or supernatural powers are needed to successfully employ these remedies. All of the procedures described in this book are safe and effective, follow the instructions without the slightest deviation. The cleansings provided are intended as *"over-the-counter"* prescriptions to be used by anyone being victimized by these agents of chaos.

ISBN 0-942272-72-2 5½"x 8½" 112 pages $9.95

TOLL FREE: 1 (888) OCCULT - 1   WWW.OCCULT1.COM